ANTI INFLAMMATORY RECIPES

Delicious Healthy Foods to Make at Home
By: Emily Simmons

Table of Contents

Introduction

Welcome, and congratulations on your purchase of a recipe book that I hope you'll use over and over in the coming days. This book aims to help you nourish your body with foods that will fight inflammation, by the use of nature's own medicines- fresh unprocessed foods, herbs, and spices.

So, who needs this book? Anyone who may be suffering from a chronic disease, as well as anyone who may wish to avoid such diseases. The book will introduce you to easily obtainable foods that you should incorporate into your diet, and will then feature them in easy to prepare, delicious recipes for you to make at home, without having to spend hours in the kitchen.

First though, we need to look at what inflammation in the body is, what causes it, and why it's not always a good thing. Since the 1980's, researchers have discovered a relationship between certain foods and certain chronic (long-term) diseases such as cancer, diabetes, arthritis, and others. They have discovered that certain foods cause inflammation in our bodies, and others calm it.

The body is actually made to use inflammation in a good way, such as to cause swelling around a wound to help seal it off, or to protect the wound from infection. However, when inflammation gets out of control, it becomes a bad thing. Sometimes the inflammatory response in the body can be so extreme that it contributes to the development of diseases such as cancer, diabetes, arthritis, and heart disease. This happens when the immune system's inflammatory response over-reacts, and instead of only attacking viruses and bacteria, or clearing out damaged cells, it starts to attack healthy cells as well.

Controlling what we eat goes a long way to controlling how our immune system will respond to threats. Different people respond differently to different foods. For example, some people feel bloated and uncomfortable after eating bread or dairy products, yet others tolerate these foodstuffs well. Some foods, however, are known to cause problems for a lot of people, and these are the ones to start eliminating from your diet first. Don't worry, though, we won't be just taking foods away from you, but we'll be making replacements with other easily tolerated, scrumptious eats. An easy way to tell what foods are best to avoid is by keeping in mind that the further removed from its natural state a product is, the more likely it is to cause inflammation in the body. (e.g. apple pie.) The closer foods are to the way they were created, the less likely they are to cause harm. (e.g. an apple.) Because of this, some of the recipes in this book are not so much recipes, as ideas for combining simple, fresh foods in a new way, sometimes without even having to cook. What could be easier than that? The way that foods are prepared also makes a difference to their nutritional value and to whether or not they will cause an inflammatory response. Deep frying your fish, for example, can change what was a health giving food into one that may cause harm. Baking it with a sprinkle of olive oil and lemon juice and a few herbs, however, keeps it tasty and retains all its nutritional value.

An interesting new finding is the role that spices and herbs can play in fighting inflammation in our bodies. Some common herbs and spices that you probably already have in your kitchen are on the list, and many have been included in the recipes which follow.

You'll want to avoid too many foods that contain omega 6's. Not because they are bad in themselves, but because our ratio of omega 3's to omega 6's should be about 1:1. Since nowadays we tend to have far more omega 3's than 6's in our diets, contributing to inflammation, we need to reduce the amount of omega 6's we consume.

BREAKFASTS

We all know that breakfast is a super-important meal, but how many of us have spare time in the morning? This chapter aims to give you ideas and recipes that are quick and easy to prepare, and that give you a boost of nutrients to get your day off to a good start. Remember, food is your body's fuel, so just as you wouldn't start a trip by filling your car with inferior quality fuel, neither should you start off your day by filling your body with inferior food.

If you stock up on fresh or frozen fruit, natural Greek yoghurt, nuts and seeds, and some eggs, you'll never be short of a quick and simple breakfast.

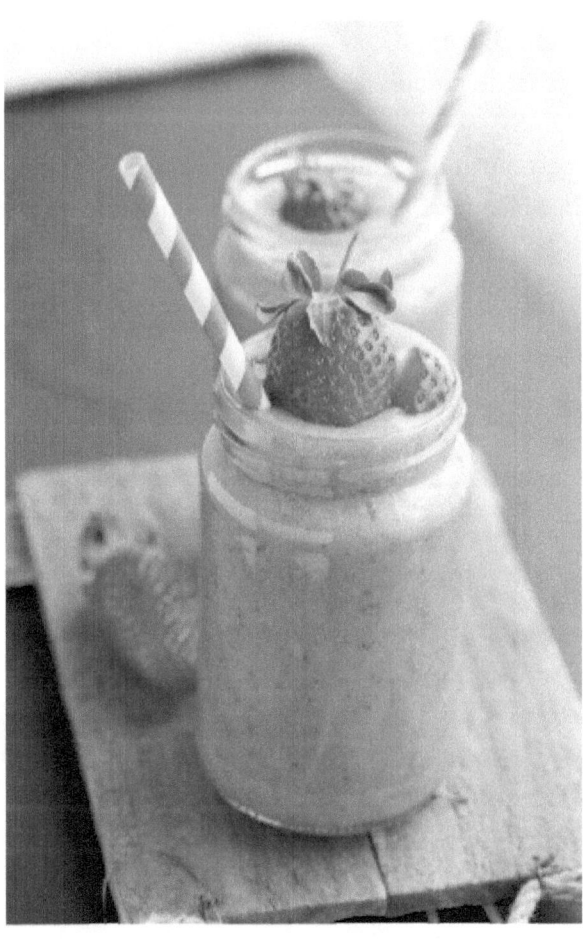

Tropical Smoothie

Making a smoothie in the morning is a really fast and easy way to pack in a lot of nutrients and hydrating liquid without having to make a huge meal.

INGREDIENTS:

½ cup coconut milk

½ cup almond milk

1 ripe banana, peeled and sliced

½ teaspoon ground cinnamon
1 tablespoon flax seeds, ground
INSTRUCTIONS:
Combine the coconut milk, almond milk, banana, cinnamon, and ground flax seeds in a blender. Blend until smooth. Pour into a tall glass and serve.

Serves 1

Passion Fruit and Blueberry Smoothie

Blueberries are among the most nutrient dense berries, and are considered a superfood. Passion fruits are rich in vitamin C. So together, they make for a really good way to begin the morning.

INGREDIENTS:

2 passion fruits, seeds scooped out into blender

1 ripe banana, peeled and sliced

1 cup fresh blueberries

2 tablespoons fresh lemon juice

1 cup plain low-fat Greek yogurt, or dairy-free milk such as almond

2 teaspoons honey

1 teaspoon cinnamon

INSTRUCTIONS:

Put the passion fruit, banana, blueberries, and lemon juice in a blender and blend together until smooth.

Add the yogurt, honey, and cinnamon and blend again.

Pour into glasses and serve immediately.

Serves 2-3

Fruit and Yogurt Meal in a Glass

Combine chunks of whatever fruit you have on hand, and make a superbly healthy breakfast in just a few minutes. Flax seeds are very high in omega 3's, and should be ground to make all the micronutrients easy to absorb.

INGREDIENTS:

1 cup plain low- fat yoghurt

A few drops of vanilla extract

½ cup fruit such as blueberries, raspberries, bananas, strawberries, or peaches, chopped into small dice

1 tablespoon flax seeds, ground

2 tablespoons walnuts, chopped

1 teaspoon honey, to serve

INSTRUCTIONS:

Mix the yoghurt and vanilla, and place half the yoghurt into a tall parfait glass. Top with half of the fruit, and sprinkle with half of the ground flax and the walnuts. Layer the remaining yoghurt on top, then the remaining fruit, nuts and seeds. Drizzle with the honey. Serve at once.

Serves 1

Pomegranate Jewel Bowls with Peaches and Yoghurt

Pomegranates are beautiful, and they've been found to have three times the antioxidants as red wine or green tea. They have potent anti-inflammatory effects, especially in diabetics.

INGREDIENTS:

1 cup fresh peaches, sliced

1/2 cup plain low-fat Greek yogurt

1 teaspoon honey

1 tablespoon flax seeds, ground

2 tablespoons fresh pomegranate seeds

Handful of almonds, chopped

INSTRUCTIONS:

Arrange the peach slices in a bowl and top with the yogurt; then drizzle with the honey.

Sprinkle with the flax seeds, pomegranate seeds, and almonds.

Serves 1

Spicy Gingerbread Oatmeal

1. This is a warm, comforting breakfast that will warm your tummy on those icy winter mornings. It's full of spices known for their anti-inflammatory effects.

1. INGREDIENTS:

1 cup steel cut oats
4 cups water
Pinch of salt
1 teaspoons ground cinnamon
½ teaspoon ground ginger
Maple syrup to taste

1. INSTRUCTIONS:
2. Put the oats, water, and salt in a saucepan and bring to the boil. Reduce the heat and simmer gently for about 15 minutes, stirring now and then. Add the spices and stir to mix. Serve the porridge hot, drizzled with maple syrup. Serve with a little milk if you like.

Serves 4

Creamy Nutty Oatmeal Porridge

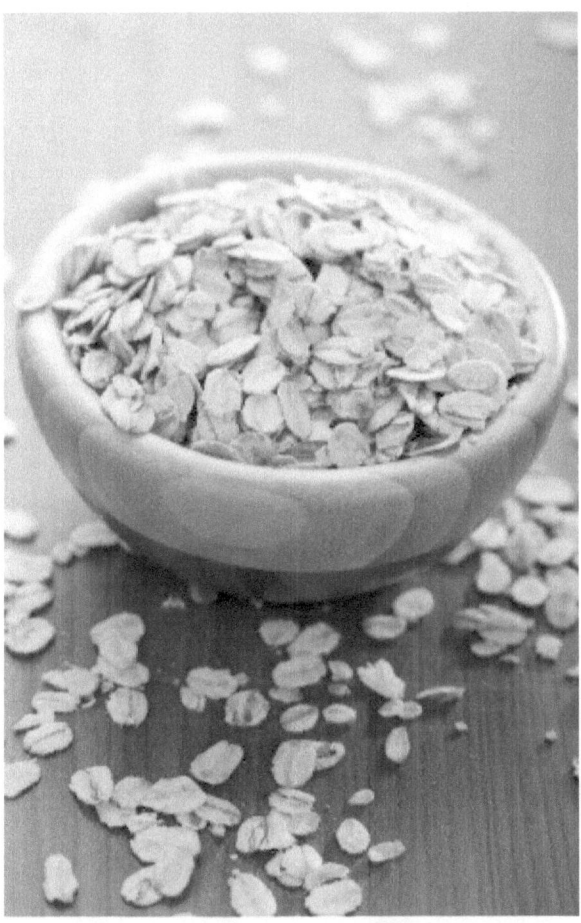

Another version of oatmeal porridge that's quick to make and provides a filling breakfast to set you up for a busy day.

INGREDIENTS:

4 cups water

1 cup steel-cut oats

Pinch of salt

1 tablespoon flax seeds, ground

¼ cup mixed raw nuts, such as cashews, almonds, or walnuts, chopped

2 tablespoons almond milk

1 teaspoon honey, or ½ teaspoon stevia

INSTRUCTIONS:

In a medium sized saucepan bring the water and oats to the boil, with a big pinch of salt. Reduce the heat to low, and simmer for about 15 minutes. Stir in the ground flax, nuts, and milk. Drizzle honey over the top. Serve hot.

Serves 1

Poached Eggs with Swiss Chard

Sometimes one just feels like a savory breakfast. Eggs are a great way to start off the day, because they're full of protein and other nutrients such as omega 3's and vitamin D. A breakfast of eggs can keep you fuller for longer and eliminate the need for a lot of snacking through the morning. An added benefit is that, for most people, eggs are anti-inflammatory. In fact, people who eat a steady breakfast of eggs, fresh fruit, and a cup of coffee can reduce their inflammation markers by up to 20 percent. It's perfectly safe to eat up to four eggs a week.

INGREDIENTS:

2 eggs

2 slices oat bread

2 teaspoons extra-virgin olive oil

1 bunch of Swiss chard, well washed, shredded

2 tablespoons chopped fresh parsley

Sea salt and freshly ground pepper to taste

INSTRUCTIONS:

Using a small frying pan, lightly stir-fry the Swiss chard in the oil until wilted and most of the water has evaporated. Season with salt and pepper.

For the eggs, bring 2 cups of water, with a teaspoon of vinegar added, to a gentle boil in a shallow pan. Break one egg into a small bowl, lower the bowl almost to the water, and tip the egg into the water. Do the same with the second egg.

Use a spoon to nudge the egg whites closer to the yolk, helping to keep the egg whites together. Leave the eggs to poach for about 3 to 4 minutes. Lift the eggs out of the water gently with a slotted spoon.

Toast the bread while the eggs are poaching. To serve, place the toast on a plate, top with Swiss chard, and then with the egg. Serve at once.

Serves 2

Sweet Potato Frittata with Tomato Relish

INGREDIENTS:

1 large sweet potato, peeled and cut into small cubes, boiled till just cooked

4 tablespoon olive oil

2 small onions, peeled and finely chopped

Sea salt and black pepper to taste

4 eggs

handful each of parsley and chives, finely chopped

3 plum tomatoes, peeled and chopped

I red chili, seeded and finely chopped

1 teaspoon agave syrup

INSTRUCTIONS:

To make the relish, heat a tablespoon of oil in a small frying pan. Fry 1 of the onions until softened, then add the tomatoes and chili. Simmer until reduced to a thick saucy relish. Season with agave, salt, and pepper. Set aside.

To make the frittata, first heat the grill (broiler) element.

Using a non-stick omelet pan (one that's ok to use under the grill) add the remaining olive oil. Heat and then add the remaining onion. Season with salt and pepper. Fry until soft, then add the sweet potatoes. Fry until golden. In a bowl, beat the eggs and pour into the skillet over the sweet potatoes. Sprinkle with parsley and chives. Cook on low heat, do not stir, until the eggs start setting. Now put the skillet under the grill to set the top. Be careful not to overcook. Loosen with a spatula and turn out onto a serving dish. Cut in half and serve at once with a dollop of tomato relish on each serving.

Serves 2

Strawberry Drinking Yogurt

For breakfast or even for when you're craving a milkshake, you're sure to love this yummy pink treat.

INGREDIENTS:

1 cup plain low-fat yogurt

½ cup strawberries, fresh or frozen
¼ cup almond milk
1 teaspoon honey or ½ teaspoon stevia
INSTRUCTIONS:
Combine the yogurt, strawberries, almond milk, and honey or stevia in a blender. Blend the ingredients until smooth and pour into a glass. Serve with a straw.
Serves 1

Cashew-Butter Toast

Making your own nut butter couldn't be easier, and it's delicious and filling on toast with honey.

INGREDIENTS:

½ cup unsalted roasted cashews

pinch of salt

2 slices oat bread

1 teaspoon honey

INSTRUCTIONS:

Combine the cashews and the salt in a small food processor bowl and puree until smooth. Toast the bread slices and spread them with the cashew butter. Drizzle the toast with honey.

Serves 1

Vegetable Breakfast Frittata

Yes, you can and should have vegetables for breakfast!

INGREDIENTS:

1 tablespoon extra-virgin olive oil

1 small onion, finely chopped

½ cup fresh vegetables, such as zucchini, spinach, broccoli, and kale, diced

2 eggs, beaten

1 tablespoon goat cheese

Salt and black pepper, to taste

INSTRUCTIONS:

Heat the olive oil in a non-stick frying pan. Sauté the onion in the olive oil for a couple of minutes until it's transparent and soft. Add the remaining vegetables and sauté for a few minutes until softened.

Pour the beaten eggs into the vegetable mixture and cook for a minute until the eggs have set. Don't stir them, just tip the pan as it cooks, lifting the edges of the egg to let the uncooked egg to trickle underneath and cook. When almost done, top with the cheese and season with salt and pepper.

Slide out gently onto a plate.

Serves 1

Mushroom Omelets with Thyme

Mushrooms provide a mineral that's not commonly found in most other fruits or vegetables- selenium. It helps the liver enzymes to function properly, and helps detoxify some cancer-causing compounds in the body. Selenium also prevents inflammation and has been shown to and also decrease tumor growth rates.

INGREDIENTS:

1 tablespoon extra-virgin olive oil

1 small onion, finely chopped

1 clove garlic, finely chopped

1 cup sliced mushrooms

2 eggs, beaten

2 goat cheese, grated or crumbled

2 teaspoons fresh thyme leaves

INSTRUCTIONS:

Heat half of the olive oil in a non-stick frying pan over medium heat. Sauté the onions and garlic until they're translucent and soft. Add the mushrooms and continue to sauté until the mushrooms are soft and the water had evaporated. Set the mushroom mixture aside in a separate bowl and keep warm. Put the rest of the olive oil into the same frying pan you used for the mushrooms, and add the eggs. Don't stir, just tilt the pan and lift the edges of the egg, letting the uncooked egg run underneath. When all the egg has almost set, spoon the mushroom mixture onto one half of the omelet, and top with the cheese and thyme leaves. Season with salt and pepper. Fold the egg over the side with the mushrooms on, and slide out of the pan onto a plate. Serve at once.

Serves 1

SOUPS

Wonderfully aromatic and satisfying, soups are probably the ultimate convenience food. They're also one of the best ways to pack a lot of nutrients into one bowl. The recipes that follow use a lot of pulses, which are high in protein and fiber, and low in fat. They also incorporate many vegetables and recommended anti-inflammatory herbs, such as celery and rosemary. So go ahead and brew a potful!

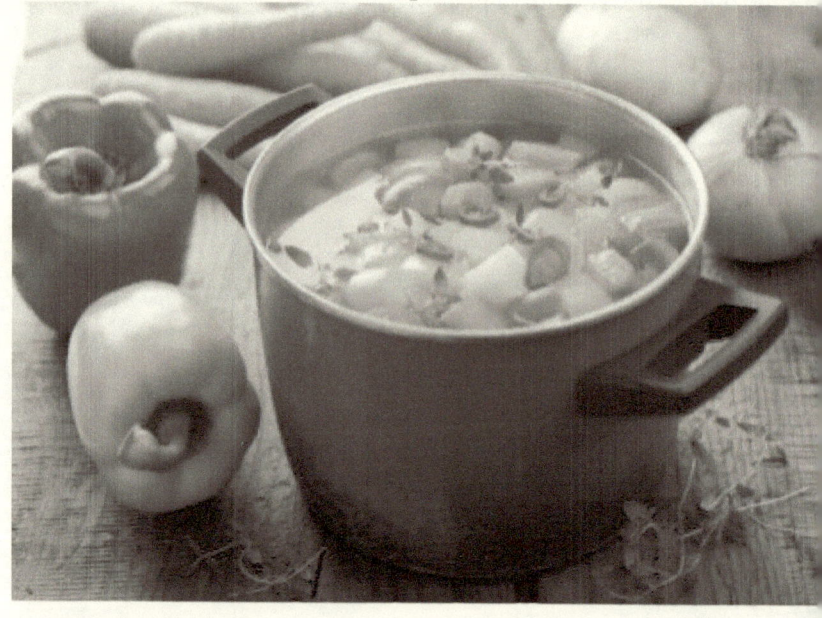

French Vegetable Soup

The addition of basil pesto at the end gives this soup a delightfully fresh flavor.

INGREDIENTS:

2 tablespoons olive oil

1 red onion, finely chopped

2 cloves of garlic, very finely chopped

1 red bell pepper, diced

1 carrot, diced

1 celery stalk, including the leaves, finely chopped

2 cups cabbage, shredded

2 tablespoons fresh oregano

2 cups kale, finely shredded

½ cup lentils

½ cup barley

2 liters vegetable or chicken stock

Handful fresh parsley, finely chopped

Sea salt and freshly ground black pepper, to taste

Basil pesto, to serve

INSTRUCTIONS:

Using a soup pot, heat the oil. Fry the onion, garlic and red pepper till softened. Add carrot, celery, cabbage, oregano, and kale. Stir fry until the vegetables have softened. Add lentils, barley and stock. Bring to a boil, then reduce heat and simmer for about an hour or until the barley and lentils are soft. Add the parsley and some salt and pepper. Serve hot, in warmed bowls, adding a teaspoon of pesto into each bowl.

Serves 8.

Barley and White Bean Soup

A substantial and nourishing soup, this is a complete meal in itself. If you don't have fresh herbs, feel free to use dried ones, only be sure to reduce the quantity.

INGREDIENTS:

2 cans cannellini beans (410g each), drained and rinsed
2 tablespoons extra-virgin olive oil
1 onion, diced
2 cloves garlic, finely chopped
2 large carrots, peeled and diced
2 cups chicken or vegetable stock
2 litres water
½ cup barley
2 sticks celery, leaves included, finely shredded
2 tablespoons fresh sage leaves, finely chopped
2 tablespoons fresh rosemary leaves, finely chopped
Sea salt and freshly ground black pepper, to taste

INSTRUCTIONS:

Using a big soup pot, heat the olive oil over medium heat. Sauté the onion, garlic, and carrots for a few minutes until softened. Add the stock, water, barley, and beans to the saucepan. Bring the soup to a boil over high heat.

Lower the heat, add the celery, sage and rosemary, and simmer the soup for about 1 hour, or until the barley is soft. Add more water as needed for the desired thickness. Season the soup to taste with salt and pepper.

Serves 6-8

Spicy Lentil and Vegetable Soup
INGREDIENTS:
2 tablespoons extra-virgin olive oil
1 onion, diced
2 cloves garlic, finely diced
1 large carrot, peeled and diced
1 teaspoon ground coriander seed
1 teaspoon ground cumin seed
½ teaspoon turmeric
2 litres vegetable or chicken stock
500g dried lentils, rinsed
½ cup mustard greens, chopped
Handful of fresh parsley, finely chopped
Juice of 1 lemon
Sea salt and freshly ground black pepper to taste
INSTRUCTIONS:
Using a large soup pot, heat the olive oil and sauté the onions, garlic, and carrot until softened. Add the coriander, cumin, and turmeric, stirring for a few seconds. Add the stock and lentils. Bring to the boil, then turn the heat down and simmer for about 30 minutes until the lentils are no longer firm. Add the mustard greens and parsley and simmer for another few minutes. Season with lemon juice, salt and pepper. Serve hot.

Serves 6-8

Golden Yellow Soup

This soup is a beautiful color, with a slightly sweet flavor. You're sure to make this again and again.

INGREDIENTS:

2 tablespoons extra-virgin olive oil

2 medium onions, peeled and diced

2 carrots, peeled and diced

1 parsnip, peeled and diced

2 litres vegetable or chicken stock

400g dried yellow split peas

1 large sweet potato, peeled and diced

1-2 tablespoons fresh oregano, chopped

Sea salt and freshly ground black pepper to taste

INSTRUCTIONS:

Using a soup pot, heat the oil and sauté the onions, carrots, and parsnips until soft.

Add the stock, split peas, sweet potato, and oregano. Bring the soup to a boil over high heat, and then reduce the heat to simmer for up to 1 hour or until all the vegetables and peas are mushy and the soup is as thick as you want. Season the soup to taste with salt and pepper.

Serves 6

Butternut and Sweet Potato Soup with Ginger

Besides being delicious, ginger is also a powerful anti-inflammatory. Some studies have shown that it's effective at reducing the symptoms of osteoarthritis, a common inflammatory disease. It has also been shown to lower blood sugars and even helps with digestion. In this smooth creamy soup, it combines well with the flavors of butternut and sweet potato.

INGREDIENTS:

2 tablespoons extra-virgin olive oil

1 medium onion, chopped

6 cups vegetable or chicken stock

1 butternut squash, peeled and cubed

1 large sweet potato

3cm piece of fresh ginger, peeled and finely grated

Sea salt to taste

1 tablespoon fresh cream per serving, to serve

INSTRUCTIONS:

Using a soup pot, heat the oil and sauté the onions until they are soft. Add the stock, butternut, sweet potato, and ginger to the pot. Bring to the boil, reduce heat and simmer for about 20 minutes until the vegetables are very soft. Allow the soup to cool for a few minutes before transferring it to a blender or food processor. Blend the soup until it's smooth. Check the seasoning. Serve in bowls with a spoonful of cream in each.

Serves 6

Pumpkin Soup with Pine Nuts

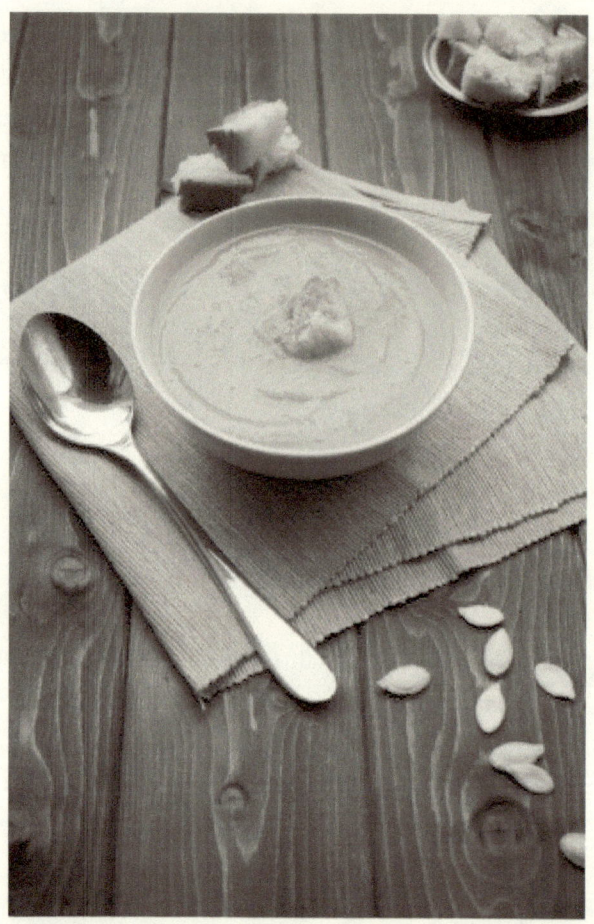

Pine nuts are a good source of vitamin E, zinc, iron, and many other nutrients. Their nutty chewiness is perfect when combined with this smooth, creamy soup, which is ready to eat in about half an hour.

INGREDIENTS:

1 ½ litres chicken or vegetable stock

1 medium pumpkin, seeded, peeled, and chopped

1 large onion, chopped

1 teaspoon ground cinnamon

2 teaspoons honey

pine nuts to serve

INSTRUCTIONS:

Using a soup pot, put the stock into it and bring to the boil. Add the pumpkin, onion, and cinnamon. Turn down the heat and simmer the soup for about 20 minutes until the pumpkin is cooked. Stir in the honey and add salt and pepper if needed. Remove from the heat and allow to cool slightly. Put it in a blender and blend or the soup until it's smooth. Return it to the pot to reheat, then serve in bowls with a sprinkling of pine nuts on top.

Serves 6

Zucchini Soup

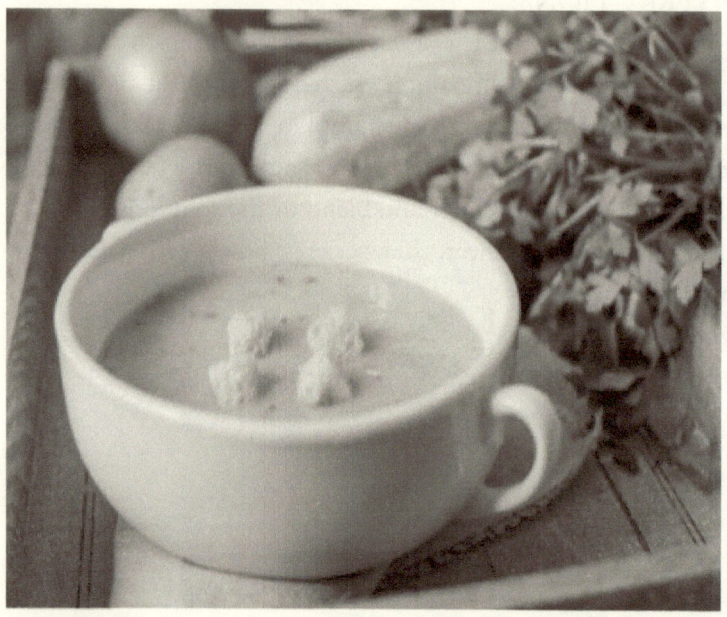

A fresh, summery soup, this is useful as a starter or it can be served as a main course with some chunky whole-wheat bread.

INGREDIENTS:

3 tablespoons extra-virgin olive oil

4 cups zucchini, grated

1 clove garlic, finely chopped

1 onion, chopped

¼ cup fresh parsley

6 cups vegetable or chicken stock

INSTRUCTIONS:

Using a soup pot, heat the olive oil over medium heat. Sauté the zucchini, garlic, and onion until they're soft. Add the parsley and stock. Bring the soup to the boil, then turn the heat down and simmer for 30 minutes. Serve hot.

Serves 8

Lentil Soup

This tasty soup provides lots of anti-inflammatory spices, and is gluten free.

INGREDIENTS:

1 tablespoon coconut oil

2 onions, peeled and finely chopped

3 cloves of garlic, crushed

1 teaspoon turmeric

1 tablespoon fresh ginger, finely grated

1 tsp ground cumin

1 tsp masala

1 teaspoon dried chili

½ tsp ground cinnamon

I large carrot, finely grated

1 cup lentils, rinsed

1 ½ cups vegetable or chicken stock

1 ½ cups coconut milk

INSTRUCTIONS:

Using a soup pot, heat the oil and fry the onion and garlic until softened. Add the turmeric, ginger, cumin, masala, chili, and cinnamon and cook for a few minutes until smelling gorgeous. Add the lentils, stock, and coconut milk. Bring to boil then reduce heat to low and simmer, uncovered, for about half an hour, or until the lentils are mushy and have absorbed most of the liquid. Serve hot.

Serves 4

SALADS

Fresh and crunchy, salads are also so quick and easy to prepare. Try having a salad every day before your main meal to help you get your nutrient quota in for the day.

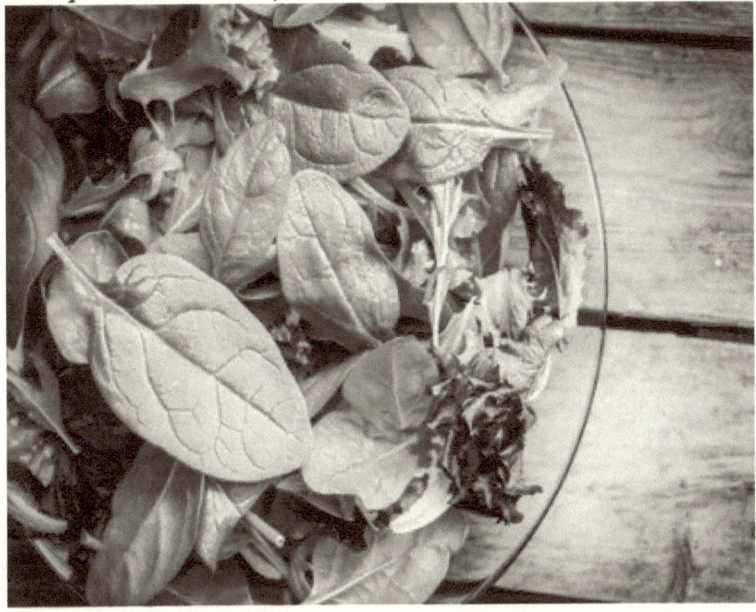

Spinach Salad with Oranges and Walnuts

To make this a complete meal, serve with a piece of lightly cooked fish, such as salmon.

INGREDIENTS:

¼ cup olive oil

¼ cup fresh orange juice

3 spring onions, white and green parts, very finely chopped

3 tablespoons white grape vinegar

1 tablespoon honey

1 teaspoon orange zest, finely grated

Salt and pepper to taste

4 medium oranges, peeled and segmented

About 180g baby spinach

2/3 cup walnuts

INSTRUCTIONS:

To make the dressing, whisk together the olive oil, orange juice, onions, vinegar, honey, and zest. Season with salt and pepper. On a serving platter, arrange your spinach leaves in a pile, then top them with orange segments. Sprinkle with the walnuts, and drizzle with the dressing.

Serves 6

Modern Cobb Salad

Always a favorite and a complete meal in itself, Cobb salad is usually very rich and full of things one shouldn't have if one is trying to eat healthily. This updated version retains all the flavor and creaminess of the classic salad, but with fewer calories.

INGREDIENTS:

Handful of salad greens
½ cup chopped broccoli
½ cup cherry tomatoes, halved
2 eggs, hardboiled and chopped
1 cup cooked, cubed turkey breast
1 large avocado, peeled, pitted, and sliced
¼ cup sliced almonds
¼ cup extra-virgin olive oil
1 clove garlic, crushed
1 tablespoon horseradish
1 tablespoons Dijon mustard
2 tablespoons red wine vinegar
Salt and pepper to taste

INSTRUCTIONS:

Use an attractive serving platter, large enough to serve 2 people. Arrange the greens first on the platter, then scatter the broccoli, tomatoes, eggs, turkey, and avocado over the top. Sprinkle with the almonds. To make the dressing, whisk together the oil, garlic, horseradish, mustard, and vinegar. Season to taste. Drizzle over the salad and serve at once.

Serves 2

Two Bean Salad

INGREDIENTS:

 1 red bell pepper, seeded, and diced
 1 green bell pepper, seeded, and diced
 1 red onion, finely chopped
 1 large tomato, chopped
 I can (about 410g) red kidney beans, rinsed and drained
 1 can cannellini beans, rinsed and drained
 1 red chili, seeded and finely chopped
 Handful of fresh parsley, finely chopped
 Juice of 2 limes
 ¼ cup extra-virgin olive oil
 Sea salt and black pepper to taste

INSTRUCTIONS:

In a bowl, mix the peppers, onion, and tomato. Add the beans, chili, parsley, lime juice, and olive oil. Season to taste. Chill and leave for a few hours before serving to allow the flavors to develop.

 Serves 6-8

Chopped Salad with Avocado Dressing

This lovely salad has a gorgeous, creamy dressing. To make it a more substantial meal, mix a can of tuna chunks into the salad ingredients.

INGREDIENTS:

1 ripe avocado, peeled, seeded, and mashed
½ small onion, grated
1 clove garlic, finely grated
Juice of 1 lemon
1 teaspoon honey
Salt and pepper to taste
½ English cucumber, diced
2 medium tomatoes, diced
Small bunch of spring onions, chopped (include some green parts)
1 baby gem or cos lettuce, shredded

INSTRUCTIONS:

To make the dressing, put the avocado, onion, garlic, lemon, honey and seasoning into a blender. Puree until smooth. If it's too thick, add a small amount of water to make a pourable dressing.

Mix all the salad ingredients together in a bowl, then tip out onto a serving platter. Top with the dressing and serve at once.

Serves 1-2

Japanese Inspired Salad

Light and refreshing, with a slight bite from the ginger.

INGREDIENTS:

1 small carrot, peeled and finely grated

2 tablespoons rice vinegar

1 tablespoon soy sauce

1 tablespoon sesame oil

1 tablespoon grated fresh ginger

1 teaspoon agave to sweeten

Handful of radishes, sliced

Handful of bean sprouts

1/3 English cucumber, peeled and halved lengthways, seeds removed and sliced

I orange, peeled and segmented

Salad greens, such as mizuna

INSTRUCTIONS:

To make the dressing, put the carrot, rice vinegar, soy sauce, sesame oil, ginger, and agave into a blender or a food processor, and process until smooth. Arrange the salad greens on a serving platter, then top with the radishes, sprouts, cucumber, and orange segments. Spoon the carrot dressing over the top and serve at once.

Serves 1-2

Spring Greens and Pineapple Salad

This salad is fresh, easily adaptable, quick to make, and it will keep well in the fridge for a few days without the dressing on. It contains the green superfoods kale and spinach, which are rich in so many nutrients, for example vitamins A, C, K, and also folic acid, and iron, to name a few. Turmeric is something we could all get more of, as it has powerful anti-inflammatory effects. With the addition of the chicken, it's a meal in itself, and a perfect lunch to take to work.

INGREDIENTS:

Bunch of kale, washed and tough center stem removed

Sea salt and freshly ground black pepper, to taste

Juice of 1 lemon

2 tablespoons extra-virgin olive oil

2 handfuls baby spinach leaves

1 handful fresh parsley, chopped

1 handful fresh mint, chopped

1 small ripe pineapple, peeled and chopped

2 handfuls raw, unbleached almonds, coarsely chopped

1 handful pumpkin seeds

2 chicken breast fillets, poached, cooled, and chopped

For the dressing:

5 tablespoons extra-virgin olive oil

1 teaspoon ground turmeric

2teaspoons freshly grated ginger

Juice of 1 lemon

1 tablespoon honey or stevia

Sea salt and black pepper to taste.

INSTRUCTIONS:

Use a large bowl. First, shred the kale with a sharp knife and place them in the bowl. Add a bit of salt and pepper, the lemon juice and oil, and leave to marinate and soften the kale for about 10 minutes. Put in the spinach, parsley, and mint. Add pineapple, almonds, and pumpkin seeds, and chicken. Add the dressing before serving, mixing it well through the ingredients. To make the dressing, whisk everything together in a small bowl until combined.

Serves 4

Crisp Clean Coleslaw

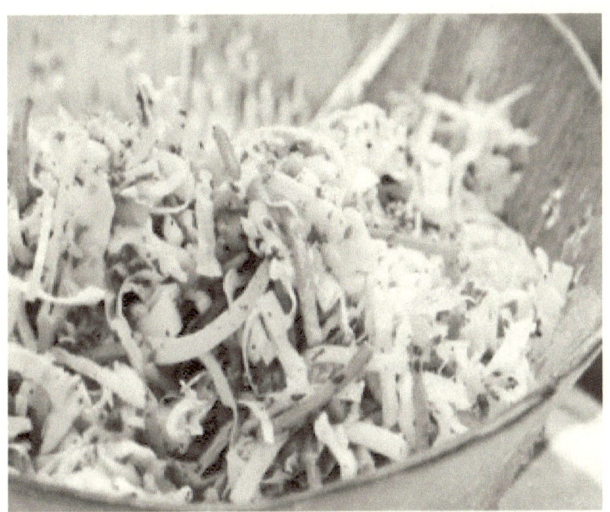

INGREDIENTS:

About 350g cabbage, finely shredded

2 large carrots, shredded

1 small red onion, finely chopped

1 green bell pepper, finely chopped

Handful fresh parsley, finely chopped

1 celery stalk, including leaves, finely chopped

Small bunch spring onions, green parts included, very finely chopped

2 tablespoons sesame seeds, lightly toasted in a dry pan

¼ cup lime juice

2 tablespoons honey

1 tablespoon apple cider vinegar

½ teaspoon ground turmeric

Sea salt and freshly ground black pepper, to taste

1 tablespoon canola oil

INSTRUCTIONS:

Using a large mixing bowl, put in the cabbage, carrots, red onion, green pepper, parsley, celery, spring onions, and sesame seeds. Mix well, using your hands. Blend the remaining ingredients together to make a dressing, tasting for seasoning. Mix into the salad and allow to stand, covered, in the fridge for about an hour before serving to allow the cabbage to soften and the flavors to blend. This salad keeps well for about 3 days in the fridge.

DINNERS

Not many of us have hours and hours after work to prepare dinner. Yet a healthy, substantial meal is still so welcome. Before you resort to unhealthy takeaways, here are some simple, fairly quick recipes that you can whip up in next to no time. It's a good idea to plan your week's menu ahead of time, so that you can buy everything ahead of time and make sure you have what you need.

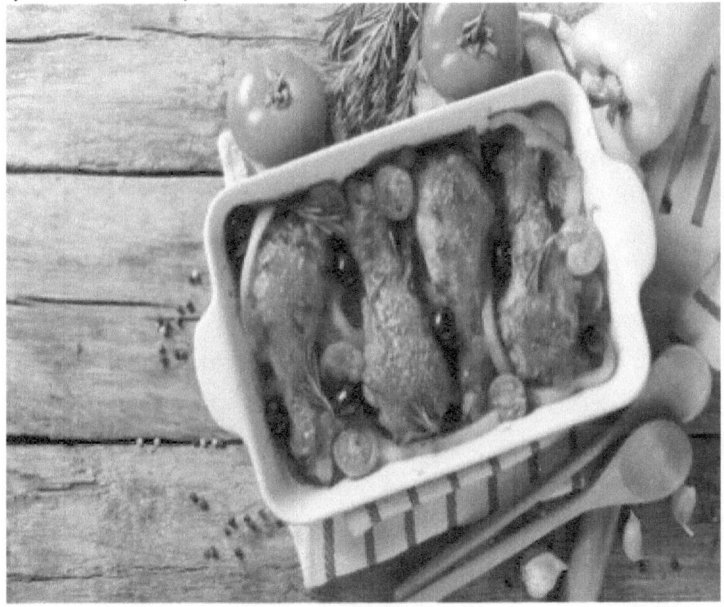

Baked Chicken

This is a wonderful all-in-one dish that can be assembled in the evening before going to bed, then refrigerating. When you come home from work the next day all you have to do is heat the oven and bake it. Miso is great for the digestion, and contains beneficial probiotics, so give it a try.

INGREDIENTS:

1½ cups chicken stock

1 tablespoon fresh thyme leaves

Juice of 2 lemons

1½ tablespoons miso paste

2 garlic cloves, crushed

1 large onion, sliced

700g sweet potatoes, sliced

5 large carrots, peeled and sliced

200g fresh green beans, topped and tailed and cut in half

6–8 organic boneless, skinless chicken breast fillets

3 tablespoons olive oil

Handful fresh parsley, chopped

¼ teaspoon cayenne pepper

INSTRUCTIONS:

Preheat oven to 220°C.

In a small bowl, mix the chicken stock, thyme, lemon juice, miso paste, and garlic. Arrange the sliced vegetables in a 3 x 22-cm baking dish. Place chicken breasts on top in a single layer. Pour stock mixture over everything, and sprinkle with the oil, parsley, and cayenne pepper. Cover with foil, shiny side facing the chicken, and bake for about an hour, turning the chicken halfway through. Serve hot with brown rice.

Serves 6.

Shrimp Pasta

INGREDIENTS:

1 tablespoon olive oil

1 tablespoon butter

1 small onion, finely chopped

1 clove garlic, finely chopped

2 medium red bell peppers, seeded and chopped

¼ cup white wine

¼ cup chicken stock

2 lemon juice

250g shrimp, peeled and deveined

200g whole-wheat pasta such as spaghetti or linguine, cooked in salted boiling water

2 tablespoons chopped parsley

A few lemon slices, for garnish

Salt and black pepper, to season.

INSTRUCTIONS:

Using a wok or large frying pan, heat the olive oil and butter. Add onion, garlic and red peppers, and sauté for a couple minutes until softened. Add white wine, chicken stock, and lemon juice. Simmer gently for a few minutes. Add shrimp, and cook for a few more minutes or until shrimp turn pink. Take off the stove, and add to the pasta, adding the parsley and seasoning of needed. Mix gently together. Serve in bowls garnished with lemon slices.

Serves 2

Thai Red Curry

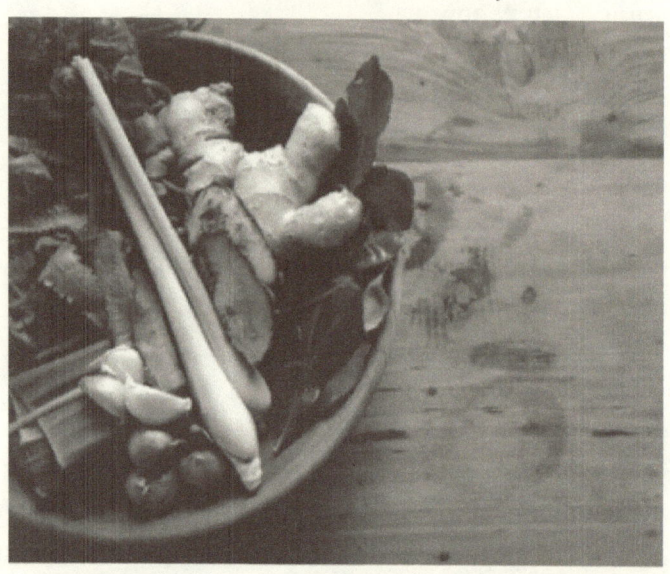

This is a delicious,exotic sounding vegetarian dish that's sure to impress any guests you may have,but is actually really easy to make.

A bonus is that it's all made in one wok, so there's less washing up afterwards! Pumpkin is highly nutritious, and is a great in
source   of   many   vitamins   and   minerals,offering beta-carotene,potassium, pro-vitamin A, vitamin C,and fiber.

INGREDIENTS:

1 ½ cups coconut milk

1-2 tablespoons Thai red curry paste, depending on how hot you like your curry

1 onion, chopped

170g pumpkin, peeled and chopped

140g green beans, chopped

1 red bell pepper, seeded and chopped

3 zucchinis, chopped

1 can bamboo shoots, drained and sliced in half

2 tablespoons fresh basil leaves, shredded

2 tablespoons lemon juice

2 teaspoons agave syrup

INSTRUCTIONS:

Using a wok, put the coconut milk, curry paste, and ½ cup water into it. Bring to the boil, stirring.

Add the onion and allow to boil for a few minutes. Add the pumpkin to the wok and simmer over medium heat until nearly cooked. Add beans, red bell pepper, and zucchini, and simmer for another 5

minutes. Add water if the sauce becomes too thick. Add the shoots and basil and carry on cooking until they're heated through. Add the lemon juice and agave syrup. Check the seasoning, adding salt if necessary.

Serve on brown rice.

Serves 6.

Curried Potatoes in Tomato Sauce with Eggs

INGREDIENTS:

900g potatoes, washed and cubed

½ teaspoon salt

2 ½ cm fresh ginger

2 cloves garlic

1 onion, finely chopped

2 tablespoon olive oil

2 tablespoons mild curry powder curry powder

1 can tomato chopped tomatoes (410g)

4 eggs

INSTRUCTIONS:

Use a large pot. Put the potato cubes in with the salt and cover with water. Bring to the boil, then simmer until the potatoes are cooked. Drain. For the sauce, peel the ginger and grate it finely. Grate the garlic too. Using a big pot or large frying pan, heat the oil. Add the onion, ginger and garlic. Sauté over medium heat for a couple of minutes, being careful not to scorch it. Stir in the curry powder, and stir until fragrant.

Add the can of tomato to the pan and stir to mix. Heat until the sauce is bubbling. Taste the sauce and add salt, if needed, and a teaspoon of honey if the tomatoes are sour. Add the potatoes to the sauce and stir to coat. Add a few tablespoons of water if the mixture seems too dry.

Create four small wells in the potato mixture with a small ladle and crack an egg into each. Place a lid on the pan and let it come up to a simmer. Simmer the eggs in the sauce for about 6-8 minutes, until cooked through (less time if runny yolks are desired). Serve immediately.

Serves 2

Turkey Bolognese

Similar to the traditional Bolognese, this take on it uses lean and healthy turkey meat instead of beef.

2 tablespoons extra-virgin olive oil

1 medium onion, finely chopped

2 cloves garlic, very finely chopped

1 large green pepper, seeded and finely chopped

1 carrot, finely grated

1 stick of celery, leaves included, finely chopped

500g lean ground turkey

1 large (790g) can tomatoes, with juice, roughly chopped

1 tablespoon tomato paste

1 teaspoon dried oregano

Salt and black pepper, to taste

1 teaspoon honey or agave

¼ cup milk

300g whole-wheat spaghetti noodles, cooked in salted water

Using a large frying pan, heat the olive oil. Add the onion, garlic, and green pepper, and stir fry till softened.

Add the carrot, celery and the turkey meat, frying until brown and breaking up the lumps as you go. Add the tomatoes, tomato paste, oregano, and seasoning. Simmer, uncovered, until the sauce has thickened and looks rich and delicious. Taste and add honey if needed to balance any sourness from the tomatoes, and add the milk for creaminess. Simmer for a further 10 minutes, and in the meantime cooking the pasta.

Serve the sauce hot over the pasta.

Serves 4-6

Roasted Chicken with Lemon, Baby Potatoes,

and Broccoli

This makes a lovely roast dinner, with minimal preparation. If you don't have fresh herbs, feel free to substitute with 1 teaspoon each of dried ones.

INGREDIENTS:

1 whole organic chicken, rinsed and dried

2 tablespoons extra-virgin olive oil plus a little more for dressing the broccoli

1 handful fresh thyme, leaves picked

1 handful fresh oregano, leaves picked

2 lemons

1 teaspoon sea salt

1 teaspoon freshly ground black pepper

1 onion, chopped

About 2 dozen new (baby) potatoes

½ cup water

4 cups broccoli spears

4 sprigs parsley, chopped

INSTRUCTIONS:

Preheat the oven to 180°C. Lightly oil a small roasting pan with half the oil. In a small bowl, combine 1 tablespoon of the olive oil with the thyme, oregano, juice from one lemon, and seasoning. Save the squeezed out lemon rind. Rub the chicken with the herb mixture and place the squeezed lemon remains in the cavity of the chicken. The rind will add flavor from the inside out. Place the chopped onion on the bottom of the roasting pan, and put the chicken on top. Scatter the baby potatoes around the sides. Cover with foil (shiny side in) and roast the chicken for an hour. Remove the foil in the last 15 min so the chicken can brown. Cook for longer if the chicken is not yet done.

While that's going on, steam the broccoli. Drain, then dress the broccoli with a little more olive oil, the juice of the other lemon, and the parsley.

Allow the chicken to rest in a warm place for 10 minutes before carving. Serve hot with the broccoli, new potatoes, and the onions from the roasting pan.

Serves 6

Cinnamon Baked Lamb with Butternut Squash

Warm and comforting, this dish is best served in fall or winter.

INGREDIENTS:

2 tablespoons extra-virgin olive oil

2 teaspoons ground cinnamon

1 tablespoon dried thyme

1 clove garlic, crushed

Salt and black pepper, to taste

4 lamb shanks

1 large onion, finely chopped

1 cup carrot dice

1 butternut squash, peeled, and cut into large dice

¾ cup water or red wine

INSTRUCTIONS:

Preheat the oven to 180°C and lightly oil a baking dish.

In a bowl, mix the rest of the oil with the cinnamon, thyme, garlic, and seasoning. Rub this mixture onto the lamb.

Put the onion, carrots, and butternut on the bottom of the baking dish. Put the lamb shanks on top of the vegetables. Pour in the water. Cover the dish with foil, shiny side facing the lamb, and cook the lamb for about an hour, or until tender, then remove the foil and cook, uncovered, for a further 20 minutes.

Serve with peas and mashed sweet potatoes.

Serves 4

Chicken and Mushroom Pilaf

Similar to a risotto, but with much less stirring! The rosemary blends so well with the earthy flavor of the brown rice and mushrooms.

INGREDIENTS:

3 tablespoons olive or canola oil

1 large onion, chopped

1 clove garlic, finely chopped

250g button mushrooms

Small handful fresh parsley, finely chopped

1 tablespoon fresh rosemary, chopped

1 ½ cups brown rice

3 cups chicken or stock

4 chicken breast fillets, cubed

INSTRUCTIONS:

Using a large saucepan over medium heat, heat half the olive oil. Add onion and garlic, and fry until softened. Add mushrooms and fry until most of their water has evaporated. Add the rice, and the stock, bring to a boil, and turn heat down to medium-low. Simmer for about 30 minutes or until stock has been absorbed. Stir now and again to prevent sticking. Add more stock if needed. Add the fresh herbs in the final 10 minutes of cooking.

Also in the final 10 minutes, heat the remaining oil in a separate pan, and fry the chicken cubes over high heat until just done and golden. To serve, mix the chicken through the rice and serve hot.

Serves 4

Salmon and Zucchini with Lemon and Herbs

This dinner is all made in one pan, so you won't have much washing up to do.

INGREDIENTS:

4 zucchinis, sliced in half lengthways

2 tablespoons olive oil

Sea salt and freshly ground black pepper, to taste
2 teaspoons agave
2 tablespoons lemon juice
2 cloves garlic, very finely chopped
1 tablespoon fresh dill, chopped
1 tablespoon fresh oregano, chopped
½ tablespoon fresh thyme leaves
2 tablespoons fresh parsley, chopped
Sea salt and freshly ground black pepper, to taste
4 (120-150g each) salmon fillets
INSTRUCTIONS:

Preheat oven to 200°C. Lightly oil a baking sheet.

Beat together the honey or agave, lemon juice, garlic, dill, oregano, thyme and parsley. Season with salt and pepper.

Place zucchini in a single layer onto the prepared baking sheet. Drizzle with olive oil and season with salt and pepper. Put salmon in a single layer on top and brush each salmon fillet with the herb mix.

Put into the oven and bake until the fish is done- when it flakes easily with a fork, which should take around 20 minutes. Serve at once.

Serves 4

Basic Stir-Fry

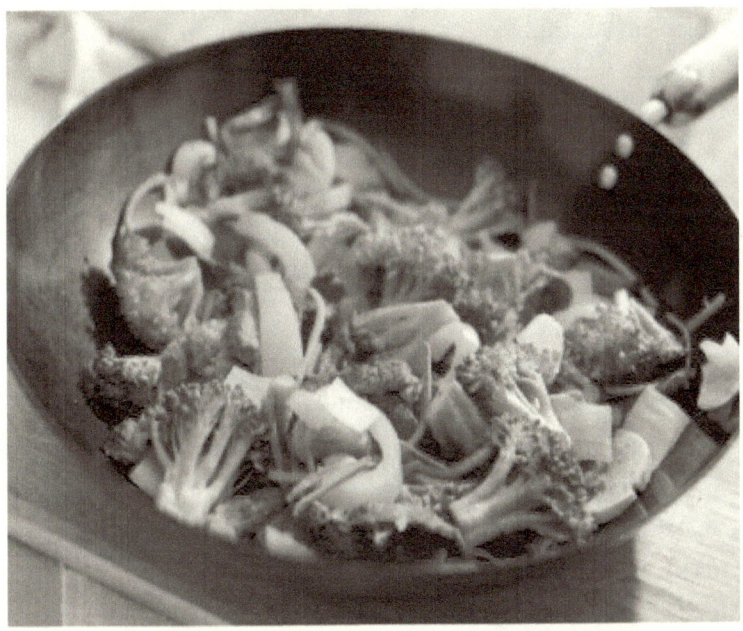

Stir fries are one of the quickest, easiest, and most nutritious meals you can make. Vary the vegetables and choice of meats each time and you'll never become tired of them.

SUGGESTED INGREDIENTS:

Vegetables such as cabbage, green beans, snap peas, bell peppers, onions, mushrooms, carrots, leeks, and zucchini.

Meats such as chicken or turkey breast, or lean pork, cut into strips (optional)

Seasonings such as soy sauce, ginger, garlic, sea salt and pepper

Oil to fry such as sesame or light olive oil.

Base to serve it on such as brown rice, gluten free noodles or rice noodles

INSTRUCTIONS:

Shred or cut all the vegetables into uniform sized strips or slices. Heat a little oil in a wok, and stir fry the vegetables until crisp-tender. Season and remove to a bowl. Wipe out the wok, add a little more oil, and stir fry the meat strips until browned. Season. Add the vegetables back to the wok and mix all together.

Meanwhile, prepare your rice or noodles. Serve with the stir-fry.

As far as quantities go, you'll need a couple of big handfuls of vegetable strips for each person, and about 100g of meat each. Remember that that vegetables reduce in volume a lot when they cook down.

Pan-Fried Salmon on Rocket Salad

INGREDIENTS:

    4 salmon fillets, about 150g each

    3 tablespoons fresh lemon juice

    4 tablespoons extra-virgin olive oil

    Salt and freshly ground black pepper, to taste

    6 cups baby rocket leaves

    1 ½ cups cherry tomatoes, halved

    2 small red onions, thinly sliced

    Salt and freshly ground black pepper, to taste

    1 tablespoon balsamic vinegar

INSTRUCTIONS:

Place the salmon fillets in a shallow dish. Pour the lemon juice and 3 tablespoons of the oil over them. Season with salt and pepper and leave to one side for 15 minutes or so.

Heat a non-stick pan on medium high heat. Pan fry the fish for just a couple of minutes on each side to sear it. Lower the heat to medium, cover the pan and cook for a further 3 minutes or so, by which point the fish should be cooked through. Don't overcook it. Set aside and keep warm.

Put the rocket, tomatoes and onions into a bowl. To serve, season the salad with salt and pepper, and dress with the remaining olive oil and the vinegar.

Serves 4

Nonna's Stew

You'll love this comforting Italian vegetable stew, which brings all the flavors of Italy right into your kitchen.

INGREDIENTS:

1/2 lb. eggplant, unpeeled and cubed

2 tablespoons extra-virgin olive oil

1 large onion, thinly sliced

3 cloves garlic, crushed

1 celery stalk, finely chopped

Handful of fresh basil, stems removed, chopped

400g can Italian tomatoes, crushed

1 tablespoon tomato paste

320g potatoes, washed and cubed

225g zucchini, cut into thick rounds

1 large red bell pepper, seeded and cubed

Salt and freshly-ground black pepper

INSTRUCTIONS:

Place the eggplant cubes in a colander with a tablespoon of sea salt. Leave it over a bowl for about 20 minutes to extract any bitter juices. Rinse under running water, drain, and pat dry.

Using a large pot, heat the olive oil. Add the onion, garlic, and celery. Stir-fry over medium heat for about 5 minutes, until the vegetables have softened. Add the eggplant, and stir-fry until beginning to stick. Add the basil and the tomatoes. When it starts simmering, add the potatoes. Stir, bring to a boil, then turn down and simmer, covered, for about 15 minutes. Add the zucchini and peppers and simmer for another 15 minutes or so, until all of the vegetables are soft.

Check the seasoning, adding salt and pepper if needed, and a teaspoonful of honey if the tomatoes are sour. Allow to sit in the warmer for 20 minutes or so before serving, to allow the flavors to develop.

Serves 4

SWEET TREATS

Yes, despite making the switch to an anti-inflammatory lifestyle, you can still have a few sweet treats now and again. Here, applesauce is used in baked goods instead of butter and too much sugar, and natural sweeteners like honey, agave, and maple syrup take care of that sweet tooth.

Strawberry Banana Frozen Yogurt

INGREDIENTS:

¼ cup almond or rice milk

3 ripe bananas, peeled and sliced

1 ½ cups fresh strawberries, sliced

½ cup plain low-fat Greek yogurt

INSTRUCTIONS:

Heat the milk in a saucepan over low heat, stirring until just warm. Take off the heat and mix in the honey. Put the bananas, strawberries, and yogurt in a blender and blend until smooth. Divide the mixture among four plastic cups. Place a plastic spoon into each one. Freeze until firm.

Serves 4

Oatmeal Cashew Cookies

INGREDIENTS:

  1 tablespoons softened coconut butter
  1/2 cup agave nectar
  1/4 cup applesauce, unsweetened
  1 egg
  1 teaspoon vanilla extract
  1 cup oats
  ¾ cup sorghum flour
  ¼ teaspoon salt
  ½ teaspoon baking powder
  ½ teaspoon baking soda
  1 teaspoon ground cinnamon
  ¼ cup cashews, chopped
  ¼ cup currants

INSTRUCTIONS:

Preheat the oven to 180°C. Prepare your cookie sheet by spraying with non-stick cooking spray, or lining with baking parchment.

Stir together the coconut butter, agave nectar, applesauce, egg, and vanilla extract.

In a separate bowl, mix the oats, flour, salt, baking powder, baking soda, and cinnamon.

Gently fold the dry ingredients into the applesauce mixture and stir until just blended. Mix in the cashews and currants. Drop heaped teaspoonfuls of dough onto the baking sheet, and flatten slightly. Bake the cookies for 10 to 12 minutes or until the edges are slightly browned. Remove from oven, allow to cool for a few minutes, then place on a wire rack to finish cooling. Store in an airtight tin.

Makes about 12

Honey-Ginger Syrupy Baked Pears

The flavors of pears and ginger go so well together, while the honey adds that extra touch of sweetness you've been craving.

INGREDIENTS:

4 ripe but firm pears, peeled, cored, and halved

4 tablespoons honey

1 teaspoon cinnamon

1-inch piece fresh ginger, peeled and grated

½ cup water

¼ cup chopped nuts, such as walnuts or cashews (optional)

INSTRUCTIONS:

Preheat the oven to 180°C. Line the base of a glass ovenproof dish with baking parchment. Place the pear halves, flat side down, into the dish. Drizzle with half the honey. Bake them for about 15 minutes or until they're soft, but not mushy.

Meanwhile, make the ginger syrup. Put the ginger, water, and remaining honey into a small pot. Bring to the boil, then simmer on medium heat for about 10 minutes until it goes syrupy. Strain. Serve warm or chilled, as you prefer. To serve, place a pear on each plate and spoon some syrup over the top. Sprinkle with cinnamon and nuts, if using.

Serves 4

Crustless Apple and Cranberry Pie

Apple pie is such a classic, and this new version is full of goodness. The apples are beautifully complimented by the cinnamon and walnuts.

INGREDIENTS:

1 egg, well beaten

¼ cup agave syrup or honey

½ cup whole-wheat flour 1 tsp. baking powder

¼ teaspoon salt

½ teaspoon ground cinnamon

½ teaspoon vanilla extract

3 cooking apples, peeled, cored, and diced

½ cup dried cranberries

½ cup walnuts, chopped

INSTRUCTIONS:

Preheat the oven to 180°C. Spray a 25cm pie dish with cooking spray.

In a large bowl, put the beaten egg, agave syrup, flour, baking powder, salt, cinnamon, and vanilla extract, and stir together well with a wooden spoon.

Add apples, cranberries, and walnuts, and mix well. Don't worry if the mixture looks lumpy. Pour into the prepared dish, and bake for 30 minutes.

Serve warm or cool.

Servings-4

Raisin and Spice Cookies

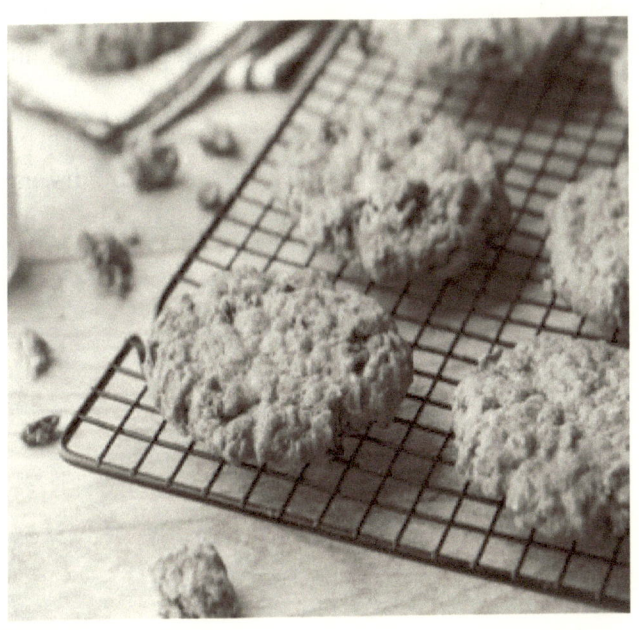

INGREDIENTS:

1½ cup spelt flour
1 cup oat flour
2 teaspoons baking powder
1 teaspoon baking soda
2 teaspoons ground cinnamon
2 teaspoons ground ginger
2/3 cup raisins
90ml coconut oil, melted
3 tablespoons rice or almond milk
1½ cups grated carrots
½ cup honey
1 egg
Pinch of salt

INSTRUCTIONS:

Preheat the oven to 180° C. Prepare a baking sheet by lining it with baking parchment, or greasing it with coconut oil.

Mix all the dry ingredients together. In a large bowl, mix all the liquid ingredients together. Add the carrots. Add the dry ingredients, mixing well. Drop with a spoonfuls onto the baking sheet and bake for about 8-10 minutes.

Makes about 35 cookies.

Oat Cookies
INGREDIENTS:
1 egg, beaten
¼ cup rice or almond milk
1 cup coconut oil, melted
½ cup honey
1 teaspoon vanilla extract
1½ cups oat flour
1 teaspoon baking soda
1 teaspoon cinnamon
1 teaspoon sea salt
3 cups rolled oats
½ cup walnuts, chopped
¼ cup sunflower seeds
½ cup apple, peeled and grated
INSTRUCTIONS:
Preheat oven to 180° C. Prepare a baking sheet by lining it with baking parchment.

In a big bowl, mix together wet ingredients. In another bowl, mix together the oat flour, baking soda, cinnamon, and salt. Mix the two mixtures together till you have a smooth batter. Add oats, nuts, seeds, and apple, stirring until combined. Drop spoonfuls onto the prepared cookie sheet, and bake for about 10 minutes.

Makes about 25 cookies.

Minty Berry Sorbet

Substitute frozen grated pineapple and mango for the berries in this dessert if you like, to make a tropical flavored sorbet, and use coconut milk instead of rice milk.

INGREDIENTS:

2 cups frozen berries, such as blueberries or strawberries

¼ cup rice milk

2 tablespoons honey or maple syrup

1 tablespoon lemon juice

Small handful of mint leaves, picked off the stem and finely chopped

INSTRUCTIONS:

Put the frozen fruit in a blender and add the rice milk. Add honey or maple syrup, lemon juice, and blend until the mixture reaches a smooth consistency. Garnish with a sprig of mint and serve at once in small dessert bowls.

Serves 4.

Conclusion

Well, it was great to end the book off on a sweet note. I hope you'll come back to these recipes again and again as you embrace a healthier way of eating.

Starting a new way of eating can seem overwhelming at first, as we are conditioned from childhood and by the culture surrounding us in a certain way. Just remember to start off slowly, making small changes in your diet one at a time, and your new anti-inflammatory way of eating will soon become a way of life that you can pass on to future generations.

You could start off by eliminating any foods that you know have a bad effect on your digestion, such as gluten or dairy, perhaps. Moving on from there, you can make small substitutions, replacing milk chocolate with dark, white bread with oat bread, and white rice with brown. You can then go on to increase your intake of fresh vegetables, perhaps cooking just one extra vegetable at dinner, or starting off dinner with a soup or a salad. Takeaway meals at lunch can then be substituted with filling salads or soup in a flask, and you'll probably find that everyone at your place of work will want some too!

After that, you can focus on breakfast, stocking up on simple fruits and yoghurt to make quick and filling smoothies, and as a contrast, having a breakfast of eggs a few times a week too.

Have a look at your drinks throughout the day, too, making sure that your main source of liquid is water. Flavor it with mint, ginger, or slices of citrus fruit if you find plain water unpalatable. Eliminate sodas and fruit punches, instead having herbal teas which come in so many flavors you're sure to find one you like. Chai teas are lovely for winter, with their warm spicy flavors they're sure to warm you up.

I wish you all the best on this journey, remember that it's a marathon not a sprint, so pace yourself and be kind to yourself, allowing for the occasional slip. After a short time, you'll start to feel the benefits, reaping the reward of increased energy, a reduction in symptoms of chronic illness you may have, fewer colds and infections, and clear glowing skin and eyes.

Enjoy the journey!